Alkaline Diet

An Exhaustive Resource On Alkaline Foods, Herbal
Remedies & Holistic Approaches For Naturally Restoring
Ph Balance, Achieving Weight Loss, And Enhancing
Overall Well-Being

Dean Clarkson

TABLE OF CONTENT

What is the Alkaline Diet

You have chosen to peruse this book due to your desire to improve your physical well-being. Your physique has been emitting indications suggesting an abnormal state of affairs. You are experiencing a suboptimal state of well-being, and you are motivated to take proactive measures to address it. The alkaline diet may potentially offer a solution to your health issues.

With the abundance of available diets, it can often become perplexing when confronted with the introduction of a novel one. Perhaps you are familiar with the alkaline diet, or have come across its name during your online investigation into methods of improving personal well-being. In the event that you possess no prior knowledge on the matter, queries may arise. Presented below are the responses.

The foundational principle of the alkaline diet rests upon the premise that our forebears adhered to a dietary regimen centered around the acquisition of sustenance from hunting and gathering. They possessed no knowledge of agricultural practices, nor did they possess access to processed and refined food products. They consumed the animals they were able to capture through hunting, while also depending on the collection of natural resources such as nuts, berries, and a variety of fruits and vegetables. They lacked grains and dairy products. They persevered and flourished, thus giving rise to our present existence. What factors would prompt individuals within the human population to modify their dietary choices in response to advancements in food production and modernization?

Our physical constitutions were not designed to tolerate certain substances that are being forcefully introduced.

The eating habits prevalent in society have produced unfavorable consequences, notably obesity and a wide range of severe and potentially fatal health conditions. The alkaline diet primarily emphasizes the consumption of food that aligns with the dietary habits of our predecessors. Nutritional items that exhibit minimal acidity and pronounced alkalinity. Reflect upon your academic years when you were enrolled in the science curriculum. Excessive acid introduction results in high acidity and low alkalinity. In the context of the human organism, this gives rise to a multitude of issues. The objective is to attain an equilibrium of the pH level, which can be accomplished by consuming an appropriate dietary regimen.

The food consumed in contemporary times often exhibits elevated levels of acidity. The alkaline diet aims to lower acidity levels and achieve equilibrium in the body's pH system through the consumption of foods that are either neutral or highly alkaline, while concurrently limiting the intake of acid-forming foods.

This dietary regimen promotes overall well-being and, as a result, it will lead to weight loss through the elimination of foods detrimental to your health and contributing to weight gain. In the following chapters, a comprehensive exploration of the manifold health advantages will be presented, alongside guidance on seamlessly integrating this dietary regimen into your personal lifestyle. This resource presents a collection of recipes that will serve as a valuable starting point for your culinary endeavors. These recipes have been specially crafted to prioritize health, while remaining easily executable and utterly delectable.

What does the alkaline diet entail?

It must be acknowledged that the Alkaline diet does not possess a substantial amount of appeal. It is alternatively referred to as the alkaline acid diet or the acid alkaline diet. This dietary approach places a significant emphasis on the consumption of fresh fruits and vegetables, tubers, as well as nuts and legumes.

The alkaline diet may not be as daunting as its name suggests, despite its stark contrast to the typical dietary choices of most individuals. It is predicated upon the consumption of minimally processed vegetation or fauna.

The concept is actually quite straightforward. It is imperative to consume dietary items that are beneficial to one's overall well-being, such as vegetables and fresh leafy greens. Conversely, it is advisable to refrain from the consumption of substances that are detrimental to one's health, such as alcohol, yeast, unhealthy fats, and sugar.

The research entails a slightly more intricate analysis than this simplified explanation. However, the primary objective is to optimize the consumption of alkaline fruits and vegetables, alongside alkaline juices and waters.

It underscores the division of alkaline foods and acidic foods, with an emphasis on the ratio of 80% alkaline foods to 20% acidic foods. This is the ratio that should be targeted. If the subject appears overly intricate, there is no need for concern because it is not. The majority of the foods we consume, after complete digestion, will either result in an alkaline or acidic state. This encompasses fish, grains, meat, shellfish, poultry, salt, and dairy products, all of which are sources of acidity commonly found in the Western diet.

While it is advisable to consume foods that have higher alkaline levels, such as fresh fruits and vegetables, this does not always prove to be the case. Consequently, our blood is characterized by a mild alkalinity, while maintaining pH levels within the normal range of 7.35 to 7.45.

The underlying principle of the alkaline diet suggests that one ought to consume a diet that corresponds to the pH level of the body, aiming for a mildly alkaline state. This is how it existed in the lives of our predecessors.

This diet represents the antithesis of the prevailing high-fat, high-protein, low-carbohydrate diets that have gained popularity. The concept of the alkaline diet and the delicate equilibrium of alkaline and acid in the body may be unfamiliar to many, but it is regularly advocated by holistic healthcare professionals and nutrition experts. It is believed that maintaining this balance is imperative for overall well-being and serves as a preventative measure against diseases such as cancer. In contrast, numerous traditional physicians hold reservations regarding the validity or endorsement of the Alkaline Diet.

What motivates individuals to embark on an alkaline diet? There is a prevailing belief that an alkaline diet can significantly alleviate chronic ailments. Presently, there exists a limited corpus of scientific evidence supporting the efficacy of this specific dietary regimen. However, it is worth noting that the diet predominantly promotes the consumption of wholesome foods, which are generally advocated by the medical community.

This dietary regimen may be beneficial for individuals who experience discomfort or adverse reactions when consuming a diet that is deficient in carbohydrates or excessive in protein. It could also prove advantageous for individuals leading demanding lifestyles and consuming excessive amounts of acidic foods.

Undoubtedly, it is advisable to consult with your healthcare professional prior to embarking on any dietary regimen. If you are afflicted with acute or chronic kidney failure, it is advised to refrain from attempting this diet without the supervision of your medical practitioner.

CHAPTER:-11

JUSTIFICATIONS FOR ADOPTING AN ALKALINE DIET

E

Everyone desires to experience a sense of well-being and achieve optimal physical functioning. If one aspires to both enhance their appearance and improve their overall state of being, the following course of action should be considered. There are three compelling rationales for making this transition: combating fatigue and low energy levels, addressing the difficulty in achieving weight loss, and ultimately, mitigating the premature effects of aging, both in terms of appearance and overall vitality.

Exhaustion and Insufficient Stamina

Numerous individuals feel fatigued and seek strategies to enhance their energy levels. Adopting an alkaline diet will prove advantageous in this regard. Strive to consume a minimum of 80% alkaline foods in proportion to 20% acid foods, thereafter gradually augment the intake of acid foods to a range of 25-30%. This will significantly enhance your energy levels compared to other conventional measures.

Weight Loss Impairment

One additional motivating factor for individuals adopting the alkaline diet is their struggle to achieve weight loss due to a need for assistance. By opting for alkaline food options such as vegetables, wheatgrass, and certain fruits like grapefruit, lemon, and lime, individuals can effortlessly attain and sustain substantial weight loss.

Additional alkaline foods include almonds (nuts), fish oil, coconut oil, flaxseed oil, liver oil, grains such as buckwheat, quinoa, and spelt, as well as condiments like sea salts, red chili peppers, and a variety of herbs and spices.

Goat's milk, beans and legumes, pumpkin seeds, and sesame seeds also serve as excellent sources for restoring alkaline balance.

It is imperative to bear in mind the importance of adequate hydration and the consumption of appropriate supplementary substances in facilitating your body's pH equilibrium.

There is currently a product available in the market known as Energy Green, which is classified as a dietary supplement. It contains numerous alkaline foods that are incorporated into its composition. Therefore, it would be unnecessary to ingest every item mentioned in the alkaline food list. All necessary components are encompassed within this single product, thus rendering it advantageous.

Premature Aging

The higher the acid levels in your body, the more your body will endeavor to adjust and restore its delicate pH balance by extracting calcium from your bones, teeth, and tissue. Calcium is one of the four alkaline elements that elevate the alkaline pH level within the human body, while simultaneously reducing the acidity levels.

There are certain experts who posit that the rapid aging process could potentially be attributed to the consumption of a significant quantity of acidic foods. Their hypothesis posits that the process of aging can be attributed to the inadequate elimination of accumulated bodily wastes and toxins.

The objective is to cease the process of aging and undo the consequences of acidic harm on the cellular structure of your body. In light of this, it is advisable to commence the process of alkalizing your body in accordance with the principles outlined in the acid alkaline diet plan. It is essential to assist your body in eliminating acidic waste.

Presented here, it is anticipated that this article has assisted numerous readers in determining the suitability of an alkaline diet for their individual needs. If you make the decision to embark upon this diet, I commend you for taking steps to enhance the quality of your life and embrace a healthier lifestyle, both for yourself and your progeny.

The Alkaline Diet Theory

In order to maintain the wellness of your body and safeguard it against ailments, it is necessary to follow a dietary regimen known as alkaline diet or acid-alkaline diet. Essentially, it is a theory positing that the consumption of food results in the production of either an alkaline or acid residue within the body, which determines its overall acid-alkaline nature, following several physiological processes such as digestion and metabolism.

The alkaline diet theory is founded upon the premise that the pH level within our organism slightly leans towards the alkaline spectrum, ranging from 7.35 to 7.45, as affirmed by certain scholarly sources stating a range of 7.36 to 7.44. Our diet should reflect this equilibrium. Any disruption in this equilibrium will give rise to significant complications within the physical system. The acidity or alkalinity of a liquid is ascertained through the pH scale. It spans a spectrum that ranges from 0 (indicating a highly acid solution) to 14 (indicating a highly alkaline solution). Seven represents the point of neutrality on the pH scale, akin to that of water. A pH value lower than 7 is indicative of acidity, which increases in strength as it decreases. Conversely, a pH value above seven represents alkaline substances, with the intensity increasing as we ascend to 14.

The scientific investigation of nearly every discipline in medicine traces its origins to the alkaline diet, although this theory is not recognized by conventional medical societies. To maintain the equilibrium of the body, it is advisable to adhere to diets featuring a 60% alkaline composition. One must adhere to highly alkaline diets (80%) due to the disruption of body balance caused by the excessive consumption of meat, eggs, cream, and other acidic foods.

When discussing alkaline diets, it is advisable to prioritize the consumption of vegetables, low-fat fruits, nuts, tubers, fresh citrus, and similar options. To enhance the body's alkalinity, fruits can be employed as a favorable resource since the majority of fruits possess high alkaline content. Only a limited quantity of fruits exhibit acidic properties. When consuming fruits for this particular objective, it is advisable to refrain from consuming canned, sweetened, or preserved fruits as their acidity levels significantly increase during the preservation process resulting from the application of various chemical agents.

In accordance with alkaline diet theory, the inclusion of vegetables is highly advised, as they serve as an excellent means of promoting alkalinity within the body. If the meat consumed for the purpose of obtaining energy becomes an acid-forming agent in the body, one may experience a sensation of weakness rather than vitality. This is because conventional medical practitioners do not perceive the consumption of vegetables as beneficial and instead insist on relying on meat consumption for obtaining energy.

Vegetables, particularly those of the green variety, serve as an excellent source for the production of alkaline compounds. These vegetables, such as carrots, cauliflower, tomatoes, and others, can be utilized in both cooked and raw forms, providing flexibility for their consumption at any desired moment. They possess a delightful flavor and offer a plethora of essential minerals. Minerals such as calcium, potassium, and magnesium serve as the principal origins of alkaline ash and are profoundly beneficial for promoting the growth and optimal functioning of the human body. Our body undergoes a transformation from an acidic state to a mildly alkaline state as these minerals interact with the acid present within our body.

Methods to Decrease Body Acidity for Enhanced Wellness

Having identified the primary factor behind acidosis and its associated challenges, we can now address it effectively to improve our overall well-being and achieve optimal physical and cognitive performance. One viable solution entails adhering to an alkaline diet, commonly referred to as an acid alkaline balance diet. The alkaline diet effectively elevates the pH level, thereby facilitating the oxygenation of body tissues and addressing both the causes and consequences of acidosis.

An optimal alkaline diet and meal plan entails abundant consumption of fresh produce such as fruits and vegetables, as well as incorporating nutrient-rich sources like nuts, seeds, and other wholesome foods. These components furnish the body with essential proteins, beneficial fats, carbohydrates, as well as a plethora of vitamins and minerals, many of which are obtainable through the consumption of fruits and vegetables in their natural state.

To achieve optimal health, it is advisable to adhere to an alkaline diet primarily composed of fresh fruits and vegetables. These will supply the body with all the necessary nutrients.

In order for the process of healing to commence, it is essential that the body maintains an alkaline state. One can mitigate the acidity of the body by incorporating a greater quantity of alkaline foods into their diet, thus facilitating the neutralization of acid levels. It is recommended that you persist with this beneficial practice until the body reaches alkalinity, thereby achieving equilibrium in the acid alkaline ratio. Upon attaining this stage, there is a regulated supply of oxygen to the cells and body tissue, leading to an enhanced immune system and the initiation of self-healing processes within the body.

Cells that are in good health possess elevated levels of oxygen and exhibit an alkaline pH. This can be accomplished by embracing a wellness regimen centered around adhering to the alkaline diet.
When the body is in an acidic state, the efficacy of symptom management for various illnesses and diseases is impeded due to the presence of an acidic environment.

The heightened acidity inhibits cellular energy production, leading to a diminished capacity for combating illnesses, diseases, and eliminating toxins in the body. Consequently, the cells become overburdened as they endeavor to eliminate the surplus acidic substances. The body experiences excessive strain and accumulates toxins within its various physiological systems.

Consequently, the body experiences fatigue and becomes susceptible to various diseases. As this repetitive cycle continues, terminal illnesses pose a significant jeopardy to one's survival.

The Alkaline Diet has demonstrated unparalleled efficacy in elevating the pH level. Pharmaceuticals, psychological strain, hazardous substances, and medical ailments hinder the efficacy of treatments by reducing the pH level.
Pathogenic conditions necessitate the presence of three essential components for their sustained growth and development:

acidity

pH levels under 6.4, indicating acidity

low oxygen

In instances where the body's acidity level increases, the pH level descends below 6.4 and concurrent oxygen levels tend to be low. This facilitates the rapid growth of bacteria, viruses, fungi, yeast, and molds. The immune system experiences a state of compromise, leading to organ malfunctions and the acidic environment suppresses the essential enzymes required for digestion.

Conditions such as cancer, Candida, cardiovascular diseases, asthma, hypertension, renal disorders, cerebral infarction, osteoporosis, arthritis, and other medical ailments thrive in such a conducive environment, defying the efficacy of any pharmaceutical interventions to impede their progression.

The presence of heightened acidity within the body is associated with the development of conditions such as osteoporosis. The human body employs an inherent mechanism whereby it endeavors to create an alkaline environment by eliminating alkaline minerals such as calcium, magnesium, and sodium from various bodily components such as muscles and bones.

Consequently, the cells counterbalance this acidic condition by expelling sodium from the stomach and mobilizing calcium from the bones, thereby triggering the initiation of rheumatoid arthritis, osteoarthritis, gout, lupus, fibromyalgia, and multiple sclerosis.

While heredity, chemical toxins, environmental pollution, and immune reactions contribute to the development of diseases such as mesothelioma lung cancer (due to asbestos inhalation), their impact is relatively limited. The prevalence of diseases is largely influenced by the consumption of an acidic diet. It is advisable to carefully monitor your dietary choices and embrace an alkaline-rich regimen consisting of a wide array of essential vitamins and minerals.

Indeed, scientific research has demonstrated that ailments are incapable of thriving within an alkaline physiological environment. Consequently, adhering to an alkaline diet assumes paramount significance in terms of promoting overall well-being, longevity, and the overall standard of living one experiences. Additionally, studies have indicated that the absence of a proper pH balance in our bodies hampers our ability to combat illnesses.

An acidic pH not only fosters the proliferation of diseases, but it also hinders the body's innate capacity to undergo natural healing processes. However, nature provides the remedy we require through the provision of unprocessed fruits, vegetables, seeds, nuts, and other nourishing foods, which can be consumed in their raw or minimally cooked state, hence supplying our bodies with essential vitamins, minerals, and nutrients essential for maintaining an optimum state of health.

The typical diet in numerous dietary plans tends to exhibit an acidic nature. It is imperative to maintain the appropriate pH equilibrium in the bloodstream, bodily tissues, lymphatic system, urinary tract, and all other bodily fluids. This objective can be accomplished by consuming a greater quantity of foods that have an alkaline effect on the body while moderating the intake of foods that contribute to acidity.

Make a concerted effort to ensure that approximately one-third of your dietary intake consists of fresh fruits and vegetables. One may incorporate alkaline-forming foods into their diet, such as almonds, apricots, raisins, dates, melons, kiwis, citrus fruits, bananas, celery, tomatoes, cherries, zucchini, and similar dietary options. Nevertheless, it is not necessary to completely eliminate acid-forming foods from your diet, as you still require a 20% intake of such foods. It is advisable to restrict their consumption and abstain from foods with little nutritional value.

Avoid

Sugar is considered acid-forming due to its chemical composition.

Soft beverages: such as carbonated drinks

The majority of grains encompass a variety of options such as wheat, wheat flour, rice, pasta, oats, barley, and others.

Animal proteins such as cow's milk, cheese, beef, eggs, chicken, mutton, pork, and so forth.

Alcohol: due to its harmful impact on cellular function in the human body. Alcohol detoxification occurs within the hepatic system. In light of an acidified body, it is advisable to alleviate the liver's burden in order to facilitate the detoxification of the acids and enable optimal energy utilization. Moreover, you do not desire the introduction of additional toxins that may impose a burden on the liver.

Coffee: due to the presence of caffeine.

Chocolate

Eat

Fruits

Vegetables with a higher level of greenness are preferable.

Assorted nuts such as hazelnuts, almonds, chestnuts, macadamia, and pecan.

Seed varieties such as sesame, flax, pumpkin, chia, and sunflower.

Nourishing fatty substances and oils: for example, flax oil, canola oil, olive oil, coconut oil.

Tofu and tempeh

Various types of herbs and spices, including but not limited to ginger, garlic, mint, basil, thyme, parsley, cinnamon, turmeric, oregano, and mustard.

Herbal teas can be utilized for the purpose of detoxification, including options such as clovers, red clover, and burdock root. Additionally, alkaline herbal teas like ginger tea, peppermint, hibiscus, and chamomile can also serve this rejuvenating purpose.

Chapter 7 - An Examination of Acidic Water

The advantages of alkaline water were previously discussed in the preceding chapter, along with the significance of maintaining a pH equilibrium, as well as the differentiation between acidity and alkalinity. However, it seems that many of us overlook a significant aspect within our alkaline water ionizer. In addition, it generates acidic water. Frequently, a query arises regarding the application of citrus water.

There are multiple applications for acid water. It can be regarded as a naturally occurring solution, as opposed to relying on the utilization of potent chemical substances. It is characterized by its environmentally-friendly nature, accommodating towards children, and additionally welcoming towards domestic animals!

The chemical water possesses disinfectant properties, making it suitable for the process of cleansing. One has the option to acquire an acidic water circulation system or collect the acid water dispensed from the Athena Ionizer garden hose, while simultaneously filling wine bottles or jugs with alkaline water.

"As previously stated, citrus-infused water contains disinfectant properties and can be employed for the following purposes:

Cleaning of the kitchen area involves washing the cutting boards, countertops (excluding marble surfaces), sinks, and other applicable surfaces. Acidic water has the potential to effectively deter infections caused by e-coli and various types of bacteria.

Promptly remove any grease from pots and pans.

Wash dishcloths and sponges. It will aid in decelerating the progression of microbes and reducing odors.

When engaging in food preparation, it is advisable to thoroughly cleanse fruits, vegetables, meats, and seafood to minimize the presence of contaminants such as E. coli and other bacterial pathogens. At your discretion, you may choose to engage in an additional wash using alkaline water.

3. Utilize the spray bottle to apply the solution as a surface cleaner or for disinfecting eyewear and refreshing the surrounding air.

Eliminate potent aromas from the hands, such as red onion or even garlic bulb! The acid water generated by your Athena Ionizer can alternatively serve as an effective hand cleanser. As a viable substitute for utilizing hand sanitizers filled with chemicals, consider using a smaller container of spray infused with solid acid water, incorporating a few droplets of your preferred essential oil, and you will be prepared.

Acidic water could also prove advantageous in the management of minor abrasions and lacerations by serving as a cleansing agent to mitigate the risk of infection. May assist in the reduction of inflammation and alleviation of pain associated with minor burns, as well as facilitate a speedy recovery.

Pustules and Dermal Pigmentation Concerns: The acidic solution generated by the ionizer possesses astringent properties that effectively manage or mitigate acne breakouts, hyperpigmentation, as well as other minor dermatological issues.

The act of purifying the body with acidic water efficaciously contributes to attaining a smooth complexion, thereby enhancing overall skin health and elasticity.

Prior to shampooing, it is advisable to cleanse the hair by rinsing it with acid water in order to mitigate the risk of hair loss, dermatitis, and scalp itchiness.

Appropriate for Utilization in the Process of Shaving. The alkaline water generated by the Alkaline Water machine aids in the management of skin irritations resulting from the process of shaving.

Furthermore, acidic water possesses potential for effectively addressing various dermatological conditions, such as:

Athlete's Foot – Can significantly expedite the recovery process, particularly when employed as a daily hot water immersion for a duration of 20-30 minutes.

Chapped Palms — May aid in the restoration of dry and cracked hands.

Insect Bites * provides alleviation from both the itching sensation and the discomfort caused by the insect bite.

To facilitate the healing process, especially when employed as a daily warm water soak for a duration of 20-30 minutes, Toenail Fungus can lend a hand in expediting recovery.

Acidic water has the potential to confer environmental benefits.

Irrigating Crops: Employ this method for the purpose of watering domestic or external crops to facilitate their growth. Plants exhibit a robust response to the application of citrus-infused water.

Aids in the preservation of freshly cut flowers when placed inside.

Promoting a pet-friendly environment, this product allows for the nourishment of your beloved household animals' skin when used for bathing purposes.

Efficient Whitening Techniques - by employing ionized citrus water, the need for hazardous chemical agents is effectively eliminated. Tidy your living space using non-chemical agents, eliminating dirt and grime while also contributing to the air's invigorating freshness.

Effectively cleans glass, mirrors, and cutlery.

The Alkaline Diet: A Guaranteed Path to Optimal Physical Well-being

To achieve the underlying causes of the illnesses, it is imperative to ensure the maintenance of an optimal pH value within our body system. Alimentary substances with inherent alkaline properties possess the capability to replenish the depleted alkalinity in the human body during the neutralization procedure. By adhering to a nutritious alkaline diet, the body is supplied with ample alkaline replenishment, thus restoring it to its predominant alkaline state.

So, what are the methods by which we can incorporate an alkaline diet into our dietary habits? The initial step is to decrease the consumption of refined dietary products. As it is widely acknowledged, the aforementioned foods are known to contain numerous chemicals that contribute to the elevation of the acidic levels within our physical constitution. The succeeding course of action involves reducing the consumption of meat and its byproducts, as well as minimizing the quantity of alcoholic beverages. The last step entails augmenting the quantity of fresh fruits and vegetables, considering their inherent high alkalinity.

Oranges and lemons are renowned for their ability to undergo alkaline conversion during digestion and are subsequently assimilated by the body as integral components of a well-balanced alkaline diet. In general, it is necessary to incorporate alkaline foods into our daily diet, accounting for approximately

75% of our total consumption. The more alkaline foods we incorporate into our diet, the more effective the neutralization of the acidic condition within our body.

Why It Is Recommended?

If you are familiar with the Atkins diet, then it can be said that the Acid Alkaline Diet stands in stark contrast to it. The Atkins diet is characterized by a significant emphasis on protein and fats, while restricting carbohydrate intake. However, these diets often result in depleted energy levels and appear to lack culinary appropriateness.

The incorporation of an acid-alkaline diet not only facilitates weight loss, but additionally, it confers substantial advantages to the physiological systems of the body. An acid-alkaline diet, also referred to as an alkaline ash diet, alkaline acid diet, and the alkaline diet, helps maintain the pH balance of the body and thus acts as a protective measure against various ailments. By adhering to such a dietary regimen, it is possible not only to prevent but also to effectively treat chronic conditions like arthritis.

The concept underlying an acid alkaline diet is rooted in the ideal pH level of our body, which should ideally be 7.3. Maintaining a slightly alkaline pH level allows for optimal functioning of vital organs and enhanced absorption of various minerals. Troubles arise when the pH of this substance tilts towards the acidic end. An elevated level of acidity in the pH results in negative effects on various bodily systems.

Given that the ideal pH value for our body is alkaline, this should be reflected in our dietary choices as well. It is recommended to increase consumption of alkalizing foods as opposed to acidifying foods. Expressed in a more formal tone, this would imply a greater focus on the consumption of vegetables and fruits, with a minimal intake of meats and oils.

When the levels of alkaline minerals, such as calcium, magnesium, and potassium, decrease within the body, its state of health will also deteriorate, leading to degeneration and a weakening of its immune defenses. An alkaline diet serves to prevent such occurrences. An acid alkaline or alkaline ash diet is composed of 80% alkalizing foods and 20% acidic foods. Given that the acid alkaline ratio in the body should ideally be maintained at a ratio of one to four, it is imperative that our dietary intake aligns accordingly.

The adoption of an alkaline diet is not solely advised for weight loss purposes, but more importantly, it serves as a significant method for reclaiming one's diminished health and attaining an extended lifespan devoid of illnesses. This particular dietary regimen is particularly recommended for individuals who frequently experience fatigue. Both stress and a reduced energy level can be alleviated through adherence to an alkaline-forming diet.

Individuals who experience recurrent viral fevers or suffer from persistent nasal congestion can enhance their overall well-being by adhering to an acid-alkaline balanced diet. Conditions such as brittle nails, dryness, headaches, muscle discomfort, allergic skin reactions, joint discomfort, and other ailments can be effectively addressed through the adoption of an alkaline ash diet.

It is advised to have an increased level of vegetable consumption within the context of an alkaline ash diet. It is recommended to extract the juice from lemons and incorporate it into water-based beverages. Millet or quinoa is preferred over wheat, olive oil over vegetable oil and soups like miso are very useful for following an alkaline ash diet.

Restoring one's physical well-being and vitality is achievable, alongside the prevention and potential cure of various persistent ailments, through adherence to an acid-alkaline dietary regimen. This diet plan is quite straightforward and has the potential to facilitate a longer and healthier lifespan for you.

Advantages of an Alkaline Diet for Individuals with Diabetes.

The human body, to a certain extent, possesses an inherent alkaline nature. By ensuring that it remains in an alkaline state, we enable it to operate at an optimal level. However, the metabolic processes in our bodies generate acidic wastes as byproducts on a vast scale. When we consume an excessive quantity of acid-producing foods and inadequate amounts of alkaline-forming foods, we exacerbate the body's acid intoxication. If we allow the accumulation of acid wastes throughout the body, a medical condition referred to as acidosis gradually develops.

If corrective measures are not promptly taken, acidosis will gradually impair our body's crucial functions. Acidosis, or excessive acidity within the body, is indeed one of the principal factors contributing to the aging process of the human body. It renders our bodies significantly susceptible to a range of severe degenerative chronic ailments, namely diabetes, cancer, arthritis, and cardiovascular conditions.

To this end, the primary obstacle confronting humanity in safeguarding our wellbeing lies in identifying the optimal approach to mitigate production while maximizing the eradication of acidic waste in the body. In order to prevent acidosis and age-related illnesses, as well as sustain optimal performance, it is imperative that our bodies adhere to a wholesome way of life.

This lifestyle should encompass regular physical activity, a well-rounded diet, a pristine physical surrounding, and a manner of living that minimizes stress to the greatest extent possible. Maintaining a healthy lifestyle enables our body to minimize its accumulation of acid waste.

The alkaline diet, alternatively referred to as the pH miracle diet, appears to be most conducive to the optimal functioning of the human body. This is primarily due to its capacity to counteract acidic waste and facilitate their elimination from the body. Individuals should consider an alkaline diet as a set of overarching dietary guidelines for individuals to adhere to.

Individuals with specific health conditions and dietary restrictions may find it more beneficial to adhere to dietary guidelines within the boundaries of an alkaline diet.

The Adoption of Alkaline Diets Contributes to the Combat Against Cancer

Over an extended period of time, alkaline diets have been purported to mitigate the likelihood of chronic ailments, including heart disease and cancer. The theory is founded upon the premise that consuming foods that align with the marginally alkaline properties of blood will result in enhanced overall well-being.

According to a source by Felicia Drury Kliment, it has been demonstrated that cancer can not only endure but also flourish within the human body, particularly when it is exposed to acidic conditions. Alkaline diets contribute to the alkalization of the body, thereby fostering the enhancement of overall well-being and fortification of the body's immune system to combat various ailments, including cancer.

The human body employs a intricate mechanism to maintain blood pH levels within an optimal range. However, the body's pH level may be disrupted and exhibit a slight acidic shift as a result of consuming specific dietary items.

In a clinical setting, it has been determined by researchers that the utilization of sodium bicarbonate may enhance the efficacy of chemotherapy agents for the treatment of cancer. Sodium bicarbonate serves as an acid buffering agent, employed for the purpose of reducing the acidity of blood under specific circumstances.

Consequently, it has been discovered that diet exerts a significant impact on the susceptibility to cancer. The recommendation to consistently consume a nutritionally balanced diet containing ample quantities of fruits and vegetables centers on maintaining the body's optimal equilibrium concerning acidity and alkalinity. The National Cancer Institute has identified cruciferous vegetables as a type of food that contains cancer-fighting compounds, among other foods. Among the assortment of vegetables present are kale, broccoli, collards, turnips, cabbage, arugula, brussels sprouts, bok choy, and cauliflower.

Alkaline therapy, also known as pH therapy, is a treatment modality for cancer developed in the 1930s, despite lacking acceptance within the mainstream healthcare sector. The treatment approach has long been regarded as an experimental or unconventional therapy.

The foundation of alkaline therapy rests upon the examination of societies with minimal cancer rates, as well as scientific scrutiny and experimentation pertaining to cellular metabolism. Based on the documented observations, it has been ascertained that the metabolic processes of cancer cells have a remarkably limited range of pH levels, specifically between 6.5 and 7.5, within which their cellular proliferation or multiplication can take place. Consequently, it is postulated that any intervention aimed at modifying the internal pH of cancer cells, either by decreasing or increasing it, holds the potential to effectively halt the progression of cancer.

Reducing the pH of cancer cells, indicative of heightened acidity, has proven to be efficacious in inhibiting cancer cell mitosis within the laboratory setting. Nevertheless, elevated levels of acidity within the human body of an individual diagnosed with cancer will impose strain upon healthy cells, thereby inducing considerable discomfort. The suggested alkaline treatment can be referred to as a 'therapy with elevated pH levels' and is intended to restore the intracellular pH balance of the patient's body by addressing latent acidosis while simultaneously raising the pH of cancerous cells to a level exceeding 7.5. Scientific investigations have demonstrated that when exposed to an alkaline pH environment, cancer cells will undergo a reversion to a regular cellular apoptosis cycle, commonly known as programmed cell death.

One frequently optimal method for pH therapy involves the implementation of an alkaline diet. The consensus among holistic practitioners and healthcare experts is that making dietary adjustments significantly aids cancer patients.

The alkaline diet effectively modifies the intracellular pH of the body to approximate the optimal blood pH level of 7.365, which is a significant metabolic achievement in pursuit of a prolonged lifespan, irrespective of an individual's cancer status. The primary focus of the alkaline diet is on plant-based foods while aiming to avoid the intake of sugar, dairy, wheat, high-gluten grains, and excessive consumption of fruits. Additionally, there is a strong emphasis on the consumption of fresh vegetables, as well as vegetable juices, particularly focusing on cruciferous vegetables and leafy greens.

The alkaline diet, consisting primarily of plant-based foods, will establish a suboptimal milieu that undermines the proliferation of cancer cells. Simultaneously, the dietary regimen will enhance the immune system and bolster the well-being of cellular structures in the body by means of enhanced nutrition.

The alkaline environment will modify the intracellular pH of cancer cells, shifting it from the preferred range for cell division (pH 6.5) to a level higher than 7.5. As a consequence, the lifespan of the cancer cells is effectively reduced. Is alkaline therapy effective for all individuals? The response is negative. Nonetheless, if the high pH therapy is administered correctly, it demonstrates efficacy in a significant proportion of individuals diagnosed with cancer. Providers estimate that approximately eighty percent of patients show a positive response to this treatment.

Achieving Optimal Performance through Adherence to the Strategy

The Alkaline Diet as a Lifestyle Choice

The alkaline diet should not be regarded as a transient endeavor, akin to a temporary weight loss regimen. Given that this diet is designed for optimizing long-term well-being rather than solely focusing on body weight, it is advisable to continue its use even when you achieve favorable medical test results and experience a general sense of well-being. What rationale exists for altering that which bestows upon you a sense of youthfulness, vitality, and overall well-being? Hence, the alkaline diet ought to be regarded as both a long-term lifestyle choice and a therapeutic measure, given its emphasis on enhancing one's overall well-being. Approximately 70% of illnesses currently recognized are attributed to dietary factors, thereby emphasizing the utmost significance of actively pursuing measures to enhance personal well-being and proactively safeguard against potential maladies resulting from suboptimal dietary practices. The alkaline diet serves as a healthful alternative to the contemporary dietary choices we make. The primary objective of this substance is to establish equilibrium between acidity and alkalinity, a complementary dynamic that could be likened to the fundamental concept of "yin and yang" within the human body.

Each health-focused dietary plan is designed with the aim of achieving somewhat similar outcomes, albeit taking distinct approaches to attain these goals. The alkaline diet has been introduced by experts to optimize bodily functions, enhance efficiency, and mitigate the risk of various ailments. This is due to the fact that the human body necessitates an optimal pH level in order for all enzymes to function properly. The maintenance of a neutral internal environment can only be achieved through the consumption of a well-rounded and nutritious diet. As the majority of food items are inherently acidic in nature, it is a common occurrence for individuals to experience conditions such as gastric acidity, indigestion, and various related ailments. The alkaline diet offers a solution to these issues by providing a proper method for regulating and balancing one's internal pH level.

The manner in which you consume your meals holds nearly equal significance to the actual content of your food. In an era characterized by hectic and demanding lifestyles, the notion of taking a well-deserved lunch break has evolved into a sought-after privilege for the majority. Engaging in brief intervals of rest while simultaneously consuming a significantly elevated volume of calories within a limited timeframe imparts a sudden impact upon the digestive system. Consuming food at a rapid pace is an unhealthy practice, as it fails to afford adequate time for the digestive system to effectively break down the food and extract all its nutritional components.

Therefore, the conventional methods by which numerous individuals consume their meals can lead to physical distortion and hinder optimal performance. These behaviors impede the body's ability to intake and utilize the essential nutrients vital for optimal bodily functions. This phenomenon gives rise to the imbalance that the alkaline diet aims to rectify.

It is imperative that individuals direct their attention towards the functioning of the human body and its requirements to restore its robustness, vigor, and vitality. By diminishing the intake of acidic food sources, such as sugars, proteins, and refined fats, and substituting them with alkaline nourishment, we initiate the initial measures towards enhancing our well-being.

The primary advantages of adhering to a prolonged alkaline diet, or adopting an alkaline diet as a long-term lifestyle, are:

Eat well

The core principles of the Eat Well philosophy revolve around the content and manner of our dietary consumption. Regrettably, we are inundated with extensively processed, commercially manufactured food products, which are abundant in added sugars, preservatives, sodium, and other substances that enhance taste. This category of food can exclusively yield adverse consequences for your overall well-being. Hence, it is imperative that we aspire to reconnect with the essence of our food, commonly referred to as "getting back to the roots". This does not imply exclusive consumption of roots (although they are beneficial for health), rather it entails the consumption of natural, unprocessed food, as it contains the necessary nutrients essential for proper bodily function, in contrast to processed food, which lacks significant nutritional content.

Live well

Merely relying on a diet, including the alkaline diet, is insufficient to guarantee enduring well-being, as it is imperative to adopt and maintain a wholesome way of life as well. The alkaline diet should be accompanied by regular physical activity. Engaging in any pleasurable activity, be it hiking, jogging, swimming, yoga, or meditation, can prove beneficial in this particular instance. One may consider practicing deep breathing techniques or engaging in cardiovascular workouts in order to enhance blood circulation, bolster physical strength, reduce stress levels, and promote a healthier overall physiological function. The presence of oxygen is indispensable for the proper functioning of the human body. Engaging in a leisurely walk outdoors to breathe in fresh air or opting to have access to it within the confines of your room is of utmost importance. These activities and factors have the potential to enhance both your physical well-being and psychological state. Arguably, music stands out as one of the most effective means of uplifting one's mood; hence, engaging in the consumption of music can greatly assist in complementing the alkaline diet.

Chapter 4: Implementation Advice

When embarking on a journey towards a state of improved well-being and opting for the Alkaline Diet as a starting point, it becomes imperative to make necessary modifications to your overall lifestyle. Certain elements of adopting a modified lifestyle may prove to be more accessible to certain individuals compared to others. If you happen to indulge in the occasional beer, it is important to be aware that the consumption of this alcoholic beverage can significantly subvert the goals you are aiming to accomplish through adherence to the Alkaline Diet. Therefore, if you are fond of consuming beer, it is imperative that you carefully deliberate upon the relative significance of your dietary requirements.

It is essential to elevate your water consumption while enhancing your dietary habits. If you do not have a predisposition for consuming water and instead prefer to quench your thirst with carbonated beverages over water, you are once again undermining the principles of the Alkaline Diet. If you are not fond of drinking water, you may wish to incorporate lemon slices as an alternative. Given that lemon is classified as an alkaline fruit, it can be utilized as a means to impart taste to your water.

Carbonated water is among the intriguing beverage options that are currently accessible. Carbonated water is available in a multitude of flavors and provides an opportunity to increase your water consumption if you have an aversion to tap water. It is advisable to carefully examine the composition of carbonated water prior to making a purchase. Numerous iterations of flavored carbonated water can be found, and several major supermarket chains stock their own labels. Nonetheless, it is imperative that you refrain from consuming beverages that contain excessive amounts of phosphates and sodium. There exists no viable substitute for ordinary water in its natural form. Nevertheless, should you come across carbonated water that contains only essential components such as carbonated water and natural flavors, you will find it devoid of any fat, sodium, or carbohydrates.

It is advisable to refrain from consuming any food items that are infused with artificial sweeteners or other synthetic ingredients. One aspect that has been observed in a society that heavily consumes processed food is our inclination towards sugary treats. Manufacturers are aware that enhancing the taste of these desserts significantly increases the probability of people consuming them and perpetuating this pattern. Their approach entails harnessing the power of your gustatory senses to work against you.

Regrettably, it is necessary to abstain from consuming coffee, teas (excluding herbal teas), and fried foods during adherence to the Alkaline Diet. It is disheartening to learn that those delectable French fries are indeed lacking in nutritional value.

It should be understood, without a doubt, that if you have not already ceased the act of smoking, it is imperative that you discontinue the usage of tobacco products. Despite their recent introduction, it is imperative that you refrain from engaging in or discontinue the use of electronic cigarettes, commonly referred to as vaping. Whilst not being derived from tobacco, the constituents engendered during the process of vaporization pose a significant risk to one's well-being.

It is advisable to actively regulate your levels of stress. The initial phase of adopting the Alkaline Diet may prove challenging, as your body may experience cravings that ultimately cannot be appeased. This will mitigate the sources of your stress. Nevertheless, by adhering to the Alkaline Diet, you will witness an amelioration in both your physical wellbeing and a reduction in your overall stress levels. As you undergo the process of eliminating acidic foods from your diet to detoxify your body, you will gradually notice the transformative effects manifesting both internally and externally.

What may come as a surprise is the manner in which your skin responds to the Alkaline Diet. Given your existing knowledge of dermal defense mechanisms utilizing acidity as a means to repel deleterious microbial intrusion, the implementation of the Alkaline Diet will facilitate an improved sensory perception and aesthetic appearance, courtesy of the buffering acidic agents present on your skin. This implies that your skin will regain its clarity and be free from any dermal issues.

Certainly, it is imperative that you engage in physical activity. There is an abundance of exercise programs accessible that will contribute to improving your overall health. Utilize low or high intensity programs that offer flexibility in the amount of effort you intend to incorporate into your regimen. As you proceed with your weight loss journey, you will notice a significant surge in your overall energy levels. You will experience reduced or minimal fatigue. Incorporating sufficient physical activity into your daily regimen will additionally enable you to shift your focus away from your cravings. You are required to rise and engage in physical activity. You will gradually recognize that reducing the burden you bear is likely to facilitate your engagement in physical activity. The increased frequency of physical activity correlates positively with an enhanced state of wellbeing. The better your physical well-being becomes, the lesser burden of stress you bear. Reduced stress levels will result in improved well-being and enhanced longevity. This way of living has a beneficial impact on your mindset.

If you opt to experiment with the Alkaline Diet, it is advisable to adhere to it for a minimum duration of two weeks. Naturally, the more time you are willing to dedicate to adhering to the diet, the more favorable the results will be. You have opted to research the Alkaline Diet. In contrast to other dietary approaches, there are no substantial demands on one's creativity. There are resemblances in this diet that bear similarities to other dietary approaches. Through the elimination of processed foods from your diet, your body will commence a recovery process, resulting in improved well-being and noticeable advantages within a month. The decision is yours to make and experimenting would not inflict any harm upon you. It is imperative to consult with a medical professional prior to commencing any dietary regimens. Maintain good health and foster clear thinking.

The Alkaline Diet Myth

Lately, there has been a considerable amount of enthusiasm surrounding the alkaline diet. Its rapid rise in popularity raises questions regarding the veracity of the abundant praise it has garnered.

It is a dietary approach that enables individuals to substitute an acid-based diet with a completely alkaline-based one.

The substitution of the alkaline-based diet with the acid-based diet has been regarded as potentially beneficial for enhancing one's overall well-being and fostering physical health.

However, conversely, it has also been asserted that this dietary approach, when substituted with an acidic regimen, effectively deters the development of cancer and substantially diminishes the likelihood of its occurrence.

Individuals have been greatly enamored and profoundly impressed by this dietary approach since its inception, paving the way for a solemn commitment to eschew all other dietary regimens for the duration of their lives.

The underlying motivation stems from their belief that incorporating this dietary regimen will enable them to achieve their health objectives with remarkable efficacy. Nevertheless, there is reason to question the efficacy of this diet and its purported ability to truly facilitate one's desired level of improvement. To ascertain the veracity, I recommend perusing this book in its entirety, which will enable you to determine its suitability for your needs.

The Liquid Diet

A liquid-based diet is a dietary plan primarily consisting of fluids, or easily digestible food items that typically liquefy at room temperature, such as gelatin and ice cream.

A liquid diet typically ensures sufficient hydration, sustains electrolyte equilibrium, and is frequently prescribed for individuals when solid food diets are contraindicated, such as for those afflicted with gastrointestinal illness or injury, or prior to or following specific types of medical examinations or procedures involving the oral cavity or the gastrointestinal tract.

Various types of liquid diets Alternative expressions: - Assortments of fluid-based dietary plans - Different varieties of liquid-centric eating regimens - Diverse selections of fluid-based nourishment plans - Various types of diets focused on consuming liquids

Transparent liquid diet

An unequivocal liquid diet consists of clear liquid nourishment, devoid of any solid particles. This includes vegetable stock, bouillon (excluding any solid remains), transparent fruit juices, transparent fruit sorbets, transparent gelatin desserts, and specific carbonated beverages such as soda and seltzer water.

The colors red and purple are strongly discouraged due to their potential to be mistaken for blood during an endoscopy or colonoscopy.

A typical menu for individuals on the prudent transparent liquid diet may bear resemblance to this.

Breakfast

1 serving of non-pulpy, unadulterated, organic fruit juice

1 dish gelatin

May I offer you a choice between espresso or tea, both of which can be served without any dairy additives?

If desired, sugar or nectar may be provided.

Lunch

1 glass of natural juice that is free of additives or preservatives

1 glass water

1 container stock

1 dish gelatin

Nibble

Complimentary frozen treat provided at no cost

One cup of espresso or tea, without any dairy additions, or a carbonated beverage.

Sugar or nectar may be added if desired.

Supper

1 container of unfettered squeezed mash or pure water.

1 container stock

1 dish gelatin

1 cup of espresso or tea, served without any dairy-based ingredients

If one desires sugar or nectar,

Comprehensive liquid-based dietary plan.

A comprehensive or restricted liquid diet consists of both transparent and turbid liquid nourishment with a smooth texture, excluding any items of crimson or violet hue. It comprises of dairy products such as milk, milkshakes, cocoa, espresso, and teas, as well as plain frozen yogurt (without any fruit, chocolate, or cookie pieces). Additionally, it includes smooth milk or dark chocolate (allowed to melt in the mouth), specific custard sweets, gelatins and puddings that are free from coconut or any other additives, strained cream soups, fruit juice with or without pulp, coconut water or coconut milk without any coconut bits or tissue, smooth cooked oatmeal such as cream of wheat (oats should be avoided due to their high fiber content). Margarine and honey are also permitted.

Water should generally be consumed based on one's thirst cues, but it is entirely devoid of nutritional value unless it is enriched with vitamins.

As a consequence of this, experts may advocate the utilization of vitamin supplements for individuals following this dietary regimen. Experts may grant specific exceptions to portions of a "restrictive" diet, such as strained meats, sour cream, cottage cheese, ricotta, yogurt, pureed vegetables or fruits, and so forth.

Lactose-free liquid diet

A lactose-free dietary regimen is a liquid diet that is characterized by its exclusion of substances containing milk or cheese.

It is commonly advised for individuals who may have lactose intolerance.

It deviates from a comprehensive liquid diet by typically excluding ice cream (including sherbet, but not milk-free sorbet), yogurt, cheese, specific creams, and any pre-prepared/pre-packaged products that may contain milk or cheese.

Reduced fiber liquid diet

A low-fiber fluid eating regimen is an eating routine that requires staying away from or bringing down substances that may contain a lot of fiber.

This dietary regimen is typically employed for individuals who are afflicted by specific gastrointestinal disorders, such as inflammatory bowel disease.

Excluded from this dietary regimen are cooked grains such as cream of wheat, oatmeal, and specific fruit or vegetable purees.

Contentions

There are a number of arguments associated with these types of diets, one of which is that they may have insufficient essential sources of nutrients to provide adequate nourishment or caloric intake, and cannot be utilized over an extended period of time.

This is largely associated with the lactose-free liquid diet, as it excludes milk, a fluid that is rich in calories, protein, and calcium. Another point to consider is that they might be lacking in dietary fiber, leading to potential gastrointestinal problems such as constipation. In certain instances, fluid weight management regimens may also induce electrolyte imbalances that can impact cardiac rhythm.

List of Liquid Diet:

Seedless organic fruit pulp or pureed organic fruit without seeds.

Vegetable extracts or blended vegetables incorporated into juices

Fluids or puréed soup with removed solids

Cooked oats that have been refined and strained, combined with a mixture of milk and cream, in equal proportions.

Gelatin without any fruit chunks.

Unadorned frozen yogurt, milkshakes, sherbet, or frozen fruit bars

Yogurt, pudding, or an intricately prepared custard

Milk or fluid nourishment supplements

Options for beverages include espresso, tea, non-alcoholic carbonated beverages, still water, or sports drinks.

Spread, margarine, or cream

Can Liquid Diets Truly Yield Results?

Fluid diets typically incorporate a decreased caloric intake, often significantly reduced. If an individual consumes fewer calories than their total energy expenditure, they will experience weight loss. On the other hand, it is possible that the diminishment in weight might be transitory.

When one significantly reduces the quantity of calories ingested, the metabolic rate decelerates in order to conserve energy. If you do not alter your dietary habits, you will regain the weight upon reverting to your previous eating regimen.

Certain dietary approaches demonstrate more effective long-term outcomes compared to others in terms of fluid weight management. Researchers have discovered that dietary regimens which encompass solid food as well as beverages can aid individuals who are overweight in managing their caloric intake during liquid meals, thus helping them sustain weight loss over an extended period.

Final Verdict:

As implied by its name, liquid weight control diets entail obtaining the majority, if not all, of your calorie intake from beverages. Certain liquid diets consist of restrictions to solely fruit or vegetable juices, or shakes, serving as replacements for the majority of your meals, consumed three or four times throughout the day.

The Influence of an Alkaline Diet on Body Weight Reduction

Over acidity in the body casues the blood to try and neutralize the acidity by pulling in alkaline salts from the bone and tissue which can lead to a whole myriad of diseases.

Foods that create acid residues in the body are:

1. Coffee

2. Black teas

3. Soft drinks or sodas

4. Meats and other flesh proteins

5. Eggs & Dairy products

6. Products that contains yeast (e.g. bread)

7. Fermented foods like soy sauce, miso, alcohol, vinegar, and sugar

The founder of this diet, Dr Young, has also found that all sugars - white and brown, maple syrup, corn syrup, high-sugar fruits as well as fruit juices, and even vegetables high in sugar like carrots and beets contributes to excess fermentation in the blood, which in turn creates excess acidity in body fluids.

A high acid content in the body fluids will in turn trigger the body to create fat to bind or hold the acidity and store it under the skin. This fat can be stored in places like our stomachs, buttocks, thighs, arms and even under our chins in order to prevent the acidity from harming our vital organs.

Acids as the name implies, will burn or erode tissue, so in essence, creating fat to store it in as to keep it from harming our bodies is in fact a life saving occurrence. While we should be thankful for it we don't need to become enslaved by it once we understand why it happens.

Once you understand this process of how your body reacts to what you eat, you can then start adopting a new way of living and eating. Changing our diet to lessen the self preservation reactions like creating fat, will lead to us having healthier, leaner more efficient bodies.

By indulging in delicious food and drinks that will not trigger the fat creation reaction,we should then be able to freely eat and drink food that will nourish our bodies, satisfy our appetites asn well as help maintain a healhty alkaline body. This way of eating is also the very best way to prevent our bodies from premature aging.

To sum it up. While the Alkaline Diet is not a diet in the traditional sense that is aimed at huge weight loss, introducing an alkalizing diet into our lives is one of the best ways to regain and to maintain an ideal weight for life.

The Alkaline Diet recommends a balance of 80/20 which means that one's diet should consist of at least 80% alkaline foods and 20% acidic foods. It is important to keep to a balance in the foods that we eat to ensure healthy bodies. Just as one will get sick if your body is too acidic, if your body is too alkaline it will also lead to getting sick.

There are many healthy foods that we can choose from to ensure that our bodies get the nourishment and energy it needs.

The Alkaline Diet lifestyle is great in that we don't need to follow extreme fad diets anymore to lose and maintain weight. Our bodies have an extraordinary capacity to heal itself. By giving our bodies food that is hydrating and asy to digest we make it easier for our immune systems to cope with the diseases that it has to fight off on a daily basis. We need to look for those foods that are most molecularly supportive in maintaining our inherent alkalinity.

Once a person has become symptom free, or once you are down to your ideal weight, then you can start reincorporating high sugar fruits and vegetables back into your diet. While these fruits and vegetables are good for you if you are healthy, in an unbalanced body it places an extra burden on the body because of their fermentation qualities.

Alkaline Diet Poached Plums

INGREDIENTS:

- 1/4 cup water
- 2 heaped tbsp. coyo coconut yoghurt
- 10 ½ oz. plums
- 1/4 tsp. agave powder
- 4 whole star anise

INSTRUCTIONS:

•Halve the plums and extract the seeds.

• Combine all ingredients in a saucepan and allow them to gently simmer over medium heat until the plums reach a soft and splitting consistency.

• Accompany with delectable syrup or with coyo coconut yogurt.

Crafting Nutrient-Dense Superfoods through the Fusion of Fruits and Vegetables

Given that the Alkaline diet mainly consists of green vegetables with limited protein and dairy, certain individuals may find it challenging to acclimate, particularly when presented with a substantial portion of greens. As a result, it is recommended to consume a portion of your vegetable consumption in its raw state. Regarding this matter, it should be noted that an alternative approach to the conventional Alkaline diet is the 80/20 split, wherein 80% of the diet consists of Alkaline foods and the remaining 20% comprises of proteins and occasional indulgences that are devoid of artificial processing or excessive refined sugars. This division should sufficiently enable the majority of individuals to restore their PH levels and consequently achieve the associated advantages.

The approach in question is commonly referred to as "juicing," a practice involving the blending of greens, fruits, and nuts to extract and unlock essential vitamins. These beverages offer a convenient means of obtaining optimal nutrition without the necessity of consuming substantial meals. It should be noted that there exists a distinction between various blenders and juicers, and it is possible that a blender may not be functional in processing food to the extent required for consuming it in liquid form. Conversely, juicers are engineered to compress and rotate the fruit, thereby extracting the entirety of its juice. One notable limitation of these juicers is that they result in the retention of the skins and certain other parts of vegetables, prompting consideration of its contents within the skin. You guessed it, nutrients. Regrettably, certain individuals are being discarded despite their potential to significantly enhance your PH level.

In recent times, a handful of machines have been introduced to the market that enhance the functionalities of both blenders and juicers. One such prominent option is the renowned "Nutri Bullet," widely recognized as the pioneering nutrient extraction device. This apparatus is capable of transforming vegetables, fruits, and nuts into a form that is highly digestible and readily assimilated by the human body. All constituents of the food undergo the process of decomposition, encompassing even the outer layers, thereby facilitating the release of essential vitamins and minerals required for optimal nutrition. It is during this process that the seeds, nuts, and fibers undergo complete pulverization, resulting in a homogenous liquid consistency that can be readily consumed without the need for extensive mastication. In addition, it alters the molecular composition of the food, thereby enhancing the process through facilitating the release of crucial nutrients.

There are numerous dietary plans available that rely on juice consumption for a certain duration, which can prove challenging for individuals as it lacks the element of physical mastication. By adhering to the principles of the Alkaline diet, one can enjoy the benefits of consuming meals at designated intervals while also availing the opportunity to enhance one's physical well-being by incorporating one or two nourishing beverages during the course of the day.

By incorporating green or natural fruit juices into your regimen, you can enhance the efficacy of the Alkaline diet and expect to experience notable improvements that may surpass your expectations, particularly within a relatively brief duration. It is noteworthy to mention that adhering to the Alkaline diet entails incorporating a significant portion of uncooked vegetables into one's dietary regimen, which presents the simplest means of achieving this objective. Therefore, you simply select your desired culinary formula, cleanse your vegetables or fruits thoroughly, and blend them together into a beverage that is entirely free of additives, rendering it both delectable and invigorating. Given the efficiency of such advanced machinery and the multitude of health benefits they offer, it is evident why these beverages are classified as superfoods. In essence, you will not only obtain all the necessary nutrients and vitamins, but these green beverages will also aid in the elimination of toxins from your body. If necessary, incorporate honey to enhance their sweetness.

Please ensure that the pH test paper is prepared for use in the morning. Once you have completed a sufficient sleep duration of six hours and prior to voiding, ensure that you have a test strip accessible. Please choose between voiding your bladder into a designated collection cup or directly onto the surface of the provided paper. The urine sample obtained immediately upon waking in the morning provides the most reliable measurement for assessing pH levels. In the event that it is not feasible to abstain from urinating for a duration of six hours, you may proceed to utilize the urine sample collected during the early morning hours. In the event of performing a saliva test, it is advised to cleanse the oral cavity by rinsing with cool water, subsequently spitting the water into the sink. Subsequently, expectorate into a spoon or a small receptacle and subsequently employ the aforementioned vessel to immerse the test paper. It is imperative to abstain from tooth brushing, eating, and drinking prior to conducting the test. Subsequently, proceed to juxtapose the examination document with the standardized color scale depicted on the packaging of the test papers. The optimal range for measuring pH in a urine test falls within 6.5 to 7.5, while in a saliva test, the preferable range lies between 7.0 and 7.5. It is worth noting that the urine test offers the most precise assessment of the body's pH level.

Upon commencing the examinations, the typical individual will exhibit pH measurements that are relatively low. This is due to the fact that the typical

American dietary pattern predominantly consists of foods that contribute to acidity within the body. The pH level can be rectified by enhancing the consumption of foods that will result in a heightened alkaline equilibrium within the human body. There is no requirement to measure the body's pH level on a daily basis. It would be highly advisable to maintain a comprehensive record of these readings through the use of a chart, as doing so would provide a visual representation of the fluctuations in the readings over a period of time.

It is of paramount importance to maintain meticulous documentation of the pH measurement during the examination of the body's pH levels. Nevertheless, it holds even greater significance to possess the knowledge and requisite understanding regarding the appropriate course of action to be taken based on those recorded readings.

The presence of pH values within the acidic range indicates that the pH of the body is more inclined towards acidity rather than alkalinity. When such an occurrence takes place, there will manifest conspicuous indications denoting an excessive acidity of the pH level within the body. In the event that the pH levels of the body become excessively acidic, individuals become increasingly prone to acquiring specific diseases and illnesses. The body is also highly likely to exhibit deficiencies in specific nutrients that play a vital role in supporting bodily functions. This exerts an avoidable burden on the physique.

The significant level of acidity present in the American diet, combined with the notable deficiency in physical exercise, readily results in an acidic body pH that falls towards the lower end of the scale. Acidosis occurs when the pH level of the body becomes significantly acidic, necessitating immediate medical intervention. This condition is rare. Typically, the pH level tends to exhibit slight acidity, yet even this mild degree can give rise to health complications that impede optimal performance in everyday activities.

There can be a multitude of issues arising, as the pH level exerts its influence on various aspects of the human physique. One experiences a pervasive sense of fatigue despite consistently obtaining a satisfactory amount of restorative sleep. The teeth and gums may experience heightened sensitivity, exhibiting bleeding or possible tooth mobility. Frequently, individuals may experience discomfort and stiffness in their neck area. The entirety of the physical structure undergoes persistent and uninterrupted discomfort, even in the absence of any discernible damage to a specific region of the body. The individual experiences recurring sinus discomfort or persistent allergies that do not subside. Headaches manifest without any discernible cause. The joints will experience persistent aching and exhibit rigidity and reduced responsiveness. Engaging in even the most minimal physical exertion results in experiencing respiratory difficulties. The process of digestion will appear to occur at a diminished pace, accompanied by recurrent episodes of either diarrhea or constipation. The individual may exhibit dermatological symptoms such as skin rashes, acne, or the onset of a yeast infection without a discernible cause. It is probable that there will be an imbalance in the hormones. Even during the balmy and humid summer months, the skin will experience a sensation of aridity. There will be a multitude of instances characterized by cognitive impairment, irritability, and depressive symptoms. Colds and other viral infections will exhibit increased frequency while their resolution may seem prolonged.

Individuals experiencing multiple symptoms listed should initiate the process of testing and monitoring the body's pH levels. If the pH levels exceed the optimal range but still do not fall into the condition of acidosis, it is likely that remedying the imbalance can be achieved through intervention at the individual's residence.

The initial measure entails reducing the consumption of processed foods. These consumables frequently possess acidity and lack any beneficial compounds for the human body. A processed food encompasses any consumable item that is pre-packaged, comprising of ingredients to which meat or other elements are added, as well as any product originating from a fast food establishment. It is recommended to refrain from purchasing any product which enumerates over four components on its packaging. The optimal nourishment for the human body entails the consumption of meals prepared using fresh ingredients within the confines of one's own dwelling.

Another crucial measure to formally embrace is the reduction or elimination of additional sugar from one's dietary intake. It is highly advisable to minimize consumption of refined sugar whenever feasible. This will certainly eradicate the consumption of carbonated beverages from one's dietary habits. In case additional sweetening is required for consumables, it is acceptable to employ stevia, unprocessed honey, or coconut crystals. Kindly ensure to employ natural sweeteners sparingly. And it is advisable to avoid the consumption of artificial sweeteners. They contribute to increased acidity levels and undermine overall well-being. The utilization of these substances frequently elicits an increased physiological inclination for greater dietary consumption.

Regrettably, individuals who consume coffee are advised to abstain entirely in cases where the body's pH level is excessively acidic. Coffee is inherently acidic and does not confer any health benefits to the body. It is advised to substitute the practice of consuming coffee with the consumption of teas or other beverages that are free from caffeine.

Although dairy products and red meat can contribute to a healthy diet, it is important to note that they can also have an acidic effect on the body. In the event of an excessively acidic pH level in the body, it may be advisable to temporarily eliminate both of these items from the dietary regime. It is advisable to incorporate additional servings of vegetables and fruits into one's diet. Thankfully, a majority of vegetables and fruits possess inherent alkalinity, thereby imparting a remarkable influence on the body's pH equilibrium. Consuming a sufficient quantity of water on a daily basis will effectively remove toxins from the body.

The body experiences adverse effects due to excessive stress and a deficiency in regular physical activity. When the human body experiences stress, the adrenal glands commence the secretion of increased quantities of two stress hormones namely adrenaline and cortisol. The excretion of these hormones prompts the body to enter a heightened state of metabolism, consequently leading to the production of surplus acid as a resultant by-product.

It is imperative to actively seek methods to minimize or eradicate daily stress to the greatest extent feasible. The disciplines of tai chi, yoga, and meditation are accessible to individuals of all backgrounds and hold the potential to alleviate the burdens of everyday stress. Adopting a predominantly inactive way of life can ultimately contribute to a rise in the overall acidity of the body's pH. The human body requires regular physical activity on a daily basis. There is no necessity for this to be more demanding than engaging in a leisurely stroll around the neighborhood after a meal. When it comes to stress relief and exercise, it is advisable to initiate at a slower pace and progressively increase the intensity. Gradually incorporate a physical fitness regimen to prevent exacerbating the pressures of an already overwhelmed existence.

Recommended Alkaline Food Choices and Foods to Steer Clear Of

It is imperative to uphold equilibrium in various dimensions of existence. Excessive abundance of a beneficial aspect can also yield negative consequences. The suggested ideal proportion of alkaline and acid ash is reputed to be 80% to 20%. If an individual can sustain such a level, it would not only revitalize their health and youth but also provide protection against a multitude of ailments. In order to endeavor and attain this ratio, it is imperative to acquire knowledge pertaining to the diverse classifications of Acid Alkaline food.

The selection of Acid Alkaline foods can be easily made when one is knowledgeable about the nature of the food. The predominant subsets of edible items that possess alkaline properties primarily consist of fruits and vegetables. Figs possess a substantially elevated level of alkaline properties. That is one of the reasons why it is advisable for individuals with health issues. The assistance of bananas in the process of healing can be attributed to the same underlying cause.

Garlic possesses excellent curative properties and is also regarded as an alkaline vegetable. Broccoli, cabbage, peas, sprouts, and nearly all vegetables are considered alkalizing foods. Individuals who desire to consume sugary substances while endeavoring to uphold their alkaline ash levels ought to contemplate utilizing stevia, as it boasts the quality of being an alkalizing sweetener in contrast to sugar.

With the exception of cranberries, all other fruits exhibit alkaline properties. Cranberries possess high levels of acidity, contributing to ash production, and therefore, excessive consumption is not advisable.

Utilizing acid alkaline food charts can effectively assist individuals who enjoy consuming meat in maintaining a harmonious equilibrium between nutritious consumption and pleasurable indulgence. By abstaining from the consumption of red meat, fish, oysters, pork, and other similar foods, an individual can effectively reduce the acidic residue present in their body.

In contrast, chicken breast is classified as an alkaline food, a classification which also applies to eggs. Upon reviewing the acid alkaline food charts, it becomes apparent as to the growing popularity of vegetarianism in contemporary times. Considering the higher alkaline ash content relative to their acidic ash, vegetarians typically incorporate a substantial amount of fruits and vegetables into their diet. Milk, however, is not advisable for individuals seeking to maintain their balanced alkaline-acid food equilibrium. Even Soymilk is acidifying.

Mineral water constitutes a crucial element in maintaining a balanced acid-alkaline diet. Water serves the dual purpose of purifying our system while also mitigating the acidic ash levels within our body.

Foods classified into the acid alkaline category are not inherently acidic or alkaline. For instance, while citrus foods possess acidic properties, their consumption ultimately leads to an alkalizing effect on the pH levels of urine.

Foods that exhibit an acidic impact on the pH of urine are referred to as acidic, in contrast to those that have an alkalizing effect on the pH of urine.

The ratio of 4 to 1 can be easily upheld when acid alkaline foods are consumed in equal proportions.

The types of food that an individual consumes can have an impact on the body's pH equilibrium. The body exhibits a higher alkaline state rather than an acidic one. It is advisable to consume foods that exhibit alkalizing properties upon undergoing metabolic processes. That is to imply they leave behind alkaline mineral residues that are utilized by the body in its various functions.

In summary, adhering to an alkaline diet aids in the prevention of the accumulation of metabolic acidity within the body, which contributes to the development of autoimmune and degenerative ailments.

Alkaline foods typically consist of natural sources such as green leafy vegetables, nuts, seeds, select fruits, and healthful oils.

In the following chapter, I have curated a compilation of the most accessible and delectable alkaline food recipes that you can incorporate into your dietary regimen to achieve optimal well-being.

Chapter 5:
The Significance of Hydration and the Vital Role of Water

You have likely received recommendations to increase your water intake. How much is enough? Water is indispensable for maintaining a proper pH balance and facilitating the process of detoxification. The choice of beverages you consume bears equal significance to your dietary choices when it comes to minimizing your toxic burden.

All substances ingested by an individual must undergo filtration and subsequently be either excreted or retained by the human body. Toxic substances impose a substantial strain on the human body, necessitating a significant exertion of our elimination mechanisms. Toxins are non-indigenous to the human body. These substances lack the ability to provide sustenance to the cellular composition of the body, thus rendering them ineffective in facilitating a healthy and vital existence.

Water is life. Water aids in the elimination of bodily waste. Water has the ability to purify, sift, and supply oxygen to our cellular structures. Drink plenty of water.

An effective method to raise the alkalinity of your body while supplying it with essential nutrients instead of depleting its alkaline reserves is through the consumption of freshly squeezed green vegetable juices. Incorporate organically grown vegetables into your juicing routine and consume the juice promptly to optimize nutrient absorption. These beverages are reliable methods to purify the body and obtain immediate vitality.

Rather than opting for that morning cup of coffee, commence your day by indulging in a rejuvenating glass of water. Alternatively, revitalizing your energy can be achieved by preparing a nutritious beverage using fresh, leafy green vegetables. By consuming a serving of freshly prepared green vegetable juice, one can enjoy sustained levels of energy throughout the day, without experiencing any periods of low energy. Additionally, detoxification can reduce the strain on your body's physiological processes.

Chapter 6:
Caffeine

Coffee is widely regarded as one of the most globally consumed and favored beverages. This is due to the energizing effects of caffeine present in coffee, coupled with the exceptionally pleasant aroma and taste offered by this beverage.

Regrettably, coffee possesses a considerable level of acidity. This disrupts the equilibrium of alkalinity and acidity. When coffee is ingested, the caffeine prompts the body to enter a state of heightened alertness, triggering the activation of the adrenal glands. This phenomenon is what engenders the sensation of heightened vitality that we all encounter subsequent to consuming a cup of coffee.

An additional principle of natural phenomenon exists, namely: objects that ascend will inevitably descend. This assertion holds validity when it comes to caffeine.

Certain individuals exhibit a higher degree of susceptibility to caffeine compared to others. Individuals who engage in the consumption of caffeine may on occasion encounter adverse effects such as headaches, depressive episodes, instances of crying, excessive perspiration, heightened anxiety, a sense of restlessness or unease, tremors, and various other manifestations associated with the sensitivity to caffeine. Other individuals are comparatively less responsive, yet they still undergo fluctuations in response to the consumption of caffeine.

Do you partake in the consumption of coffee? Do you depend on caffeine as a means of sustaining your energy throughout the day, only to find yourself waking up fatigued once more? Do you regularly find yourself compelled to reach for subsequent servings of coffee, perpetuating an unending cycle in your pursuit of the elusive state of sustained vitality?

Coffee is a stimulant. It yields temporary results. If one consumes coffee with the purpose of gaining energy, one must inevitably confront the subsequent episodes of diminished energy. That is the inherent characteristic of stimulants.

They induce bodily stimulation and generate transient surges of energy, yet these elevated states are ultimately succeeded by periods of diminishing vitality.

Caffeine is not the sole food stimulant. Sugar elicits a comparable physiological response within the human body. Upon abstaining from coffee and sugar, I experienced a sudden awareness of inner tranquility. I ceased to experience significant levels of anxiety towards circumstances that had previously overwhelmed me. I discovered that I could effortlessly reach decisions without experiencing distress or bewilderment.

I was astonished by the notable shift in my overall disposition in the absence of caffeine. I initially attributed these symptoms to my personality, but it was ultimately discovered that the presence of coffee (and sugar) in my diet was the underlying cause of my anxiety, mood swings, and depression.

Farewell coffee, greetings to genuine and, most significantly, enduring vitality.

2. "Dieting and The Alkaline Diet: A Comparative Analysis

A diet encompasses all substances ingested by the human body, whether in the form of liquids or solids, which may include carbohydrates, proteins, vitamins, and starches. It is important to note that anything consumed by the human body as a means of providing energy and fortitude contributes to the concept of a diet. Throughout the course of your life, it is highly probable that you have become accustomed to diverse dietary regimens, such as the well-balanced diet, which essentially comprises a suitable amalgamation of proteins, carbohydrates, starches, and vitamins in a single meal. Nevertheless, there exists a variety of dietary approaches, including the alkaline diet, that merit attention. The alkaline diet, as its name implies, consists of a medley of fruits, vegetables, and beverages that possess inherent properties for balancing acidity within the body. It is imperative and obligatory to adhere to the alkaline diet; one need only consider the testimony of patients within a hospital setting to find widespread agreement in this regard.

Advantages of adhering to an alkaline-based dietary approach

Aids in the regulation of blood pH balance.

Enhances mineral content within our bloodstream, such as calcium, which promotes dental health, phosphorus... and so forth.

Aids in the elimination of toxins from the body.

Facilitates the enhancement of skin formulation, resulting in improved skin health and increased pigment enrichment.

Serves as a viable alternative to commercially produced oil due to its diverse array of constituents, including the avocado fruit which contains abundant amounts of natural fats.

Aids in the prevention of ailments such as hypertension, gastric ulcers, malignancy, and diabetes.

There are numerous additional benefits to adhering to an alkaline diet, as it is one of the dietary approaches aimed at rejuvenating the body to its inherent physiological equilibrium.

Ramifications and indicators of inadequacy or complete absence of alkaline activity within the body.

Foods with alkaline properties, including avocadoes, beetroot, and other similar items, aid the body in attaining a balanced acid-base equilibrium by counteracting excessive acidity present in the blood cells and bodily tissues. By achieving this equilibrium, the body can effectively regulate acid levels and maintain optimal pH, resulting in enhanced resistance to a range of diseases.

Acne, a prevalent dermatological condition, manifests as the presence of rough, indurated skin often accompanied by the formation of papules or pustules.

Acidosis, commonly known as the kiss of death disease, denotes a condition characterized by the presence of elevated levels of acidity within the human body. The majority of the concentration is located within the body tissues and circulatory system. Failure to address this issue disrupts cellular activities and processes, subsequently leading to additional ailments. One such condition is unexplained fatigue - a state of exhaustion experienced without exertion.

High blood pressure. In the majority of instances, elevated blood pressure, characterized by heightened blood flow force, is frequently instigated by inadequate consumption of alkaline food substances, resulting in high acidity levels within the body. Consequently, this leads to an augmented heart rate, thereby imposing greater pressure.

Obesity, characterized by an inability of the body to efficiently metabolize dietary fat, cholesterol, starches, certain carbohydrates, and some proteins, results in bodily enlargement due to inadequate breakdown and neutralization of cholesterol acids in the absence of adequate alkaline essentials.

Additional manifestations of alkaline deficiency encompass vomiting, discolored urine, gastrointestinal distress, impaired cognitive function, coughing, perplexity, and somnolence.

Additional illustrations of alkaline foods comprise but are not limited to: broccoli, celery, cucumber, eggplant, garlic, ginger, and numerous other varieties.

Further information regarding the alkaline diet can be obtained from a qualified nutritionist in your vicinity or a knowledgeable vendor specializing in the sale of fresh produce.

Now that you have acquired comprehension regarding the components and principles of an alkaline diet, it is appropriate to embark upon a brief instructional session intended to initiate practical application. Assemble the aforementioned constituents and proceed to create a fruit-based beverage, such as a juice or cocktail, or alternatively, engage in the preparation of a dessert. A straightforward recipe for an alkaline juice would consist of either grape juice or lemon juice. Presented herein are a selection of culinary recipes for your consideration. These guides encompass dishes that are straightforward in their preparation and possess an element of enjoyment in their creation.

Nutritional Supplements

Consuming dietary supplements can facilitate the maintenance of a slightly alkaline state within your body, akin to the principles advocated by the alkaline diet. While you are consuming a considerable amount of nutritious food, there are specific dietary supplements that can aid in the process of alkalizing your body.

We shall proceed with enumerating several supplements that are commonly employed by adherents of the alkaline diet. Nonetheless, it would be prudent to seek advice from a medical practitioner or a healthcare expert prior to incorporating them into your dietary regimen.

Green Powder

Typically, these powders comprise a composite of chlorella algae or spirulina, alongside extracts derived from wheat, barley, or alfalfa grass (frequently, a blend encompassing all the aforementioned elements). Upon inspecting the components, one may experience a sensation akin to imbibing a concoction reminiscent of stagnant marsh liquid. Nevertheless, when mixed with a cup of water or incorporated into a smoothie, the green powders reveal a remarkably palatable flavor that is sure to please.

Regarding their health benefits, they possess the ability to enhance the alkalinity of your body, thereby affording you additional vitality and fortifying your immune system. There is a wide variety of green powders that are available in the market, and you will undoubtedly discover the suitable option for your needs. Nonetheless, ensure that you select a reputable manufacturer that has received positive feedback.

Calcium

When the internal pH levels of the body lean towards acidity, the organism initiates the process of extracting minerals from various sources, including the skeletal system. If there is a consistent depletion of calcium from your bones, they will acquire a susceptibility. Calcium is among the minerals that hold potential value for enhancing bone structure and density when consumed in the form of supplements. Regarding the daily range, it fluctuates among individuals, although the recommended daily intake falls within the range of 800 to 1500 mg, as per the RDA (recommended daily allowance).

Magnesium

In the context of acidity, the phenomena affecting your muscles is analogous to that occurring in your bones. The sole disparity lies in the fact that magnesium sustains your muscle mass and strength. Contrary to popular belief, statistical findings indicate that a staggering 75% of individuals endure a deficiency in magnesium. If you frequently experience muscle tension or headaches, it may be prudent to investigate magnesium as a potential contributing factor. The utilization of mineral supplements may prove beneficial. The suggested daily dosage falls within the range of 400 to 800 mg.

Powders and Droplets for pH Adjustment

In addition to traditional supplements, there are specifically tailored formulations aimed at promoting the equilibrium of your internal pH levels. These products are available in the market under the names "pH powder" or "pH drops," or similar appellations. Typically, these powders and drops contain a solution composed of hydrogen peroxide or chlorine dioxide. These substances possess the capacity to liberate oxygen within your body, facilitating the restoration of optimal pH levels. Furthermore, these supplements may also encompass the inclusion of essential minerals like calcium, magnesium, and potassium.

The issue at hand is that the quality exhibits significant variation contingent upon the manufacturer or the constituent components. When selecting pH powders or drops, it is advisable to undertake diligent research on the manufacturer and thoroughly read the product label.

I have now covered all the recommended supplements that

individuals following the alkaline diet should consider incorporating into their routine. We would like to reiterate that it is imperative to seek guidance from a medical practitioner prior to commencing the use of any new dietary supplements.

White Processed Vinegar

Despite expectations, vinegar is typically considered to have an alkaline nature. Nevertheless, it is important to note that white processed inexpensive vinegars tend to exhibit high levels of acidity, and for this reason, it is advisable to refrain from using them.

Other Sources:

Besides food, there are other ways to unintentionally acidify yourself.

One is through medications. Regular consumption of a significant quantity of aspirin is likely to result in the maintenance of a low pH level. This does not imply that you should completely abandon the use of aspirin, particularly if it is incorporated in a preventative healthcare regimen aimed at reducing the risk of heart-related issues. Nevertheless, if the decision to take aspirin remains discretionary, it may be advisable to discontinue its usage.

Tobacco has the characteristic of being acidogenic as well. Smoking cigarettes poses numerous detrimental consequences, not least of which is the acidification of your body.

Your pH levels may become acidic due to exposure to specific chemicals, such as herbicides. Nevertheless, there is a dearth of research to reference in connection with this matter. (It is advisable not to expose yourself to ROUND UP in any case.)

Debatable:

There is a certain degree of uncertainty surrounding the acidity or alkalinity of certain products. As an illustration, mustard is frequently mentioned as encompassing both options. As is vinegar.

Generally, the factors contributing to this phenomenon are often related to the utilization of food processing techniques or the incorporation of chemical additives that have the potential to induce acidity. Hence, white vinegar exhibits greater acidity in contrast to organic brands of Balsamic or cider vinegar which may possess alkaline properties. Another example is mustard. Commercially available yellow mustard typically possesses a higher acidic content in comparison to certain varieties of high-quality horseradish or Dion mustard, which tend to exhibit a more significantly alkaline nature.

Balancing the Alkalinity

Now, let us examine the various categories of food that can effectively reduce the elevated levels of acidity in your body.

Alkaline Fruits

While certain types of fruits possess a slight acidic composition, such as tomatoes, there exist others that exhibit a distinctly alkaline nature. The fruits that warrant consideration include: MANGO, MELONS, PAPAYA, CANTALOUPE, KIWI, APRICOTS, APPLES, RIPE BANANAS, DATES, RIPE BANANAS, WATERMELONS, and select varieties of berries (acai presents a favorable option).

Several of these fruits are particularly notable. As an illustration, a watermelon possesses a pH level of 9 and serves as an exemplary cleansing agent. You may also opt to consume watermelon juice as a standalone beverage to quench your thirst, while simultaneously promoting alkalinity within your body.

"Acid" Fruit

When considering the concept of alkalinity, does the association of limes and lemons come to mind? Traditional beliefs may imply that these substances possess acidity, however, contrary to popular belief, they possess a remarkable level of alkalinity. The pH level of a lemon exhibits a significantly high alkalinity, measuring at 9.0. While lemon juice demonstrates acidic properties, it genuinely acts as an electrolyte. One example of the potential benefits of lemon juice is its ability to restore optimal pH levels in individuals experiencing gastrointestinal discomfort, specifically heartburn caused by excessive stomach acid production. It is advisable to ensure the availability of lemons for the majority of the recipes mentioned in this book. If this method proves effective for that particular dish, consider enhancing its alkalinity levels by adding a dash of lemon.

Cinnamon

Cinnamon originates from the bark of the perpetual cinnamon tree. It serves various culinary functions, and is regarded as among the most alkaline spices. Cinnamon is frequently incorporated into subsequent recipes to impart bursts of alkaline flavor. Furthermore, as elucidated in my literary work entitled NATURAL WEIGHT LOSS HACKS AND SECRETS REVEALED, cinnamon possesses intriguing properties due to its capacity to enhance metabolic activity. A heightened metabolic rate equates to

Coconut

Frequently, you will encounter coconut ingredients listed as a versatile alkalizing indulgence. One notable aspect of coconuts is their wide range of applications. The oil can be utilized for cooking purposes, the meat serves as a wholesome vegetarian protein source, and the milk can be employed as a substitute for conventional milk in vegan culinary preparations.

Curry

Popular spice across Asia. Curry is a versatile ingredient that can be incorporated into a wide range of culinary preparations. It is possible to purchase it in powdered form and utilize it to create unique sauces.

Garlic

Highly alkaline and highly beneficial for numerous other reasons. An exemplary method for savoring the flavor of garlic is by delicately roasting a clove, sliced in half, within an oven set to a temperature of 400 F for a duration of 15 to 20 minutes. The caramelized garlic possesses a pleasant sweetness and has the potential to serve as a delectable condiment.

Mushrooms

Japanese Shiitake mushrooms have been found to possess an alkalizing impact.

Leafy Green Vegetables

Leafy green vegetables will constitute a significant source of alkalinity in this diet. The alkaline nature observed is attributable to chlorophyll, an inherently alkaline compound. The inclusion of appropriate green substances in your diet also entails the incorporation of crucial nutrients such as vitamins K, A, C, E, dietary fiber, vitamin B2, magnesium, iron, folate, among others.

You should think about:

ASPARAGUS: Derived from asparagines, an amino acid known to contribute to cognitive capabilities. This particular botanical specimen exhibits an exceptional level of alkaline content.

BROCCOLI: Exceptionally flavorful whether gently cooked or consumed fresh in its raw state. Highly alkaline.

SPINACH: Convenient to acquire, exquisite in a multitude of culinary preparations. Significant quantities of all essential nutrients, as well as being a reliable natural source of calcium.

Kale, a highly touted dietary ingredient that receives extensive attention in my literature focused on combating aging and achieving weight loss through natural means. Irrespective of the diet you may opt for, whether it is this one or an alternative, it is advisable to make kale an essential part of your everyday nutritional intake. That singular factor will have a substantial impact.

AVOCADO: An abundant source of beneficial fats, alkaline properties, and essential nutrients provided by nature.

Prepare a mashed avocado by incorporating the juice of a lemon, resulting in a simple yet delightful snack option. It can also be employed for the creation of imaginative culinary concoctions. One may also consider incorporating it into pies, blending it with pumpkin, to create a delightful green pumpkin pie.

Peppers

Upon examination, it will become evident that numerous alkaline recipes are often enriched, whenever feasible, with peppers. This encompasses a variety of peppers, which span from fiery chili peppers to the more widely consumed and potentially less challenging bell peppers in different hues, such as green, red, yellow, and orange. Additionally, peppers offer a plethora of health benefits. The crimson, golden, and tangerine-hued bell peppers possess abundant carotenoids, which play a crucial role in promoting skin well-being and have been observed to inhibit the progression of aging.

Sea Salt

Despite sodium exhibiting acidic properties, this phenomenon can be attributed, to some extent, to the chemical transformations that occur during the processing of common table salt. In contrast, it can be observed that natural sea salt possesses a higher alkalinity. This information is highly valuable as certain food items may lack palatability without the addition of salt. Consequently, you have the option to substitute your conventional table salt and sodium-containing processed foods accordingly. The optimal source of alkaline salt would be pink Himalayan rock salt, readily available at various specialty grocery stores.

Are PH levels truly hazardous?

Indeed, that is correct! An excessively acidic or alkaline pH environment is detrimental to various entities, particularly the human body. Just as acid rain is capable of ravaging a forest and alkaline waste can contaminate a lake, an imbalanced pH gradually erodes all bodily tissues, steadily deteriorating the 60,000 miles of our veins and arteries, much like corrosive substances progressively erode marble. In the absence of intervention, an unsettled pH level will impede the normal cellular processes and operations within the body, encompassing vital functions such as the rhythmic pumping of the heart and the neural impulses essential for brain function... An asymmetrical pH disrupts the equilibrium essential to all forms of existence.

It is imperative for your body to uphold its internal pH within a highly restricted range. A well-functioning body ensures sufficient alkaline reserves to counterbalance the acidity and effectively maintain its pH level. The body experiences a state of weakened condition due to the depletion of alkaline reserves, caused by the need to neutralize excessive acidity. In accordance with numerous experts, maintaining a diet that is balanced in terms of pH levels is an essential factor in preserving the requisite resources for the maintenance of good health. It is advisable to conduct a pH testing in order to ascertain the pH levels of your body and assess whether immediate attention is required. Through the utilization of pH test strips, one can swiftly and effortlessly ascertain their pH level within the confines of their personal residence. If the morning urinary pH level ranges from 6.0 to 6.5, and the evening urinary pH level ranges from 6.5 to 7.0, it indicates that your body is operating within a favorable range of functionality. Should the pH level of your saliva maintain a consistent range of 6.5 to 7.5 throughout the entirety of the day, it indicates that your body is operating within an optimal state of health. The optimal time for assessing your PH levels would be approximately one hour prior to consuming a meal, as well as two hours following the completion of a meal. The pH level of the body's fluids is regulated primarily by the abundance of water, which constitutes approximately 70% of the human body. The body maintains a pH level, referred to as the acid-alkaline or acid-base ratio, which represents a state of equilibrium between ions with positive charges (acid-forming) and ions with negative charges (alkaline-forming). The body constantly endeavors to achieve a harmonious pH balance. When the equilibrium is disrupted, a myriad of issues can arise. As the pH decreases, the acidity of the solution increases, whereas as the pH increases, the alkalinity of the solution becomes more pronounced. A neutral solution exhibits neither acidity nor alkalinity, indicating a pH value of 7.

What affects PH?

Insufficient water intake is a prevalent cause of debility and exhaustion. The consumption of water can invigorate an individual in a similar manner to how a dehydrated plant rejuvenates upon being placed in water. In order to comprehend the manner in which water can contribute to enhancing your energy levels during midday hours, it is imperative to gain insight into the mechanisms governing the pH equilibrium within your body. Typically, the kidneys regulate our electrolyte concentrations, including calcium, magnesium, potassium, and sodium. When confronted with acidic substances, these electrolytes are employed for the purpose of countering acidity. Elevated levels of acidity compel our physiological systems to extract minerals from the skeletal structure, cells, organs, and tissues. Cells ultimately face a deficiency of minerals, leading to insufficient ability to effectively eliminate waste or facilitate complete oxygenation. The absorption of vitamins is hindered by the depletion of minerals.

Harmful substances such as toxins and pathogens tend to build up within the body, resulting in a decline in the efficiency of the immune system.

The blood's pH exerts a significant impact on all bodily systems, and the organism employs various mechanisms to regulate the acid-base equilibrium of the blood. The body actively regulates the acid-base equilibrium of the blood, as even slightest deviations from the established norm can significantly impact the functioning of crucial bodily elements such as the brain, arteries, heart, muscles, and various organs. It has the potential to engender systemic overload, thus precipitating severe ailments such as cancer. The majority of dietary patterns engender an unfavorable acidity level. Indeed, the pivotal determinant in upholding optimal pH levels throughout the body appears to be one's dietary choices. Scientific findings indicate that when the process of food metabolism occurs, it produces specific chemical and metallic remnants referred to as a noncombustible \\\"ash\\\". This ash, upon interacting with our bodily fluids, generates either acidic or alkaline properties of pH. Certain foods exhibit an acidic nature, while others possess alkaline characteristics. These foods can be referred to as acid-forming and alkali-forming respectively. The majority of foods that are rich in protein (such as meat, fish, poultry, and eggs), as well as nearly all carbohydrates (including grains, breads, and pastas) and fats, have the tendency to generate acidity in the body. Conversely, most fruits and vegetables have an alkalizing effect. It is worth noting that although certain fruits, like oranges and grapefruit, contain organic acids and possess an acidic taste, they do not contribute to acid formation during metabolism, leaving no acidic remnants. In a similar vein, it should be noted that Free Form Amino Acids do not possess acidogenic properties. Rather, they possess distinctive buffering capabilities that aid the body in counterbalancing the accumulation of acidic wastes. One method you can employ to record the disparity following the adoption of a more diet that promotes alkaline production is by measuring the duration of breath retention. Adhering to a mindful eating regimen can prove beneficial. If you have excessively high acidity levels, consider augmenting your intake of fruits and vegetables. If you exhibit high alkalinity, it is recommended to augment the intake of foods that promote acidity. It would be prudent to contemplate implementing a water system that effectively filters your tap water while also producing alkaline water. The presence of elevated lead levels in potable water is a matter of utmost importance to public health. It exposes adults to potential health hazards, including but not limited to cancer, stroke, kidney disease, cognitive impairments, and hypertension. Children are inherently more susceptible to potential harm owing to the fact that their bodies, which are still in the midst of rapid growth, tend to assimilate the contaminant at an accelerated pace.

Consequently, what is the significance of the abbreviation PH in relation to water? Essentially, the pH value serves as a reliable indicator to discern the hardness or softness of water. The pH level of distilled water is measured at a neutral value of 7. Typically, water possessing a pH below 7 is widely regarded as acidic, while water with a pH above 7 is commonly categorized as alkaline. The typical pH values observed in surface water systems fall within the range of 6.5 to 8.5, while groundwater systems generally exhibit a pH range between 6 and 8.5. Alkalinity signifies the water's ability to resist a shift in pH towards acidity. It is imperative to assess the alkalinity and pH levels in order to ascertain the corrosive properties of the water.

Copper, Iron, Zinc, and Manganese are additionally classified as secondary drinking water contaminants. It is probable that these contaminants will result in the presence of hard water and the occurrence of staining issues within residential settings. However, if detected at heightened concentrations, they have the potential to result in a range of health complications. This encompasses symptoms such as nausea, emesis, dysentery, abdominal discomfort, nephropathy, and hepatopathy.

ALKALINE RECIPES

In the event that the aforementioned foods do not align with your current dietary preferences, or if you seek assistance in promoting bone health, I have some exceptional recipes that you may consider trying:

Avocado-licious

Avocado smoothie

Cocoa-infused blended bowl

Avocado crema

Almond forward

Smoothie infused with almond butter

Tamari almonds

Zoodles with almond butter dressing

Banana loaded

Cacao and banana smoothie

Smoothie made with banana and oatmeal.

Banana-based ice cream alternative

Root vegetable gathering" or "Root vegetable soiree

Salad consisting of vegan taco ingredients

Tortilla with potatoes

Smoothie made with cherry beet

Watermelon-y deliciousness

Watermelon smoothie

Smoothie made with summer melon

Watermelon popsicles

Cucumber fresh

Blended beverage made with fruits and vegetables

Beverage to alleviate bloating

Smoothie for enhancing digestion

The recipe provided below for smoothie cubes is an excellent one as it incorporates various alkaline vegetables.

WHAT ABOUT ALKALINE WATER?

Investigations conducted in Japan revealed that regular consumption of alkaline electrolyzed water led to enhanced general well-being and exercise performance among individuals who were in good health. Although numerous scientific studies were inconclusive regarding the favorable impacts of consuming alkaline water, a single study demonstrated the potential of alkaline water in alleviating symptoms associated with acid reflux.

Formula for Preparing Alkaline Smoothie Cubes

Numerous individuals have encountered improvements in their health by augmenting the consumption of alkaline foods and increasing their intake of water in their diets. Scientific research indicates that the influence of food on the pH levels in the bloodstreams of healthy individuals is negligible. However, this research also highlights the absence of alkaline foods in a well-rounded diet. Thus, augmenting one's consumption can result in a state of contentment and optimal physical well-being.

This recipe incorporates a variety of alkaline vegetables with alkaline water. Thoroughly mix all ingredients until fully combined, and subsequently transfer the mixture into a freezer tray. After solidifying, dispose of these cubes into a freezer bag and store until they are required.

If you are prepared to incorporate these cubes, I suggest substituting 4 of them with the leafy green component in your upcoming smoothie. While incorporating these nutrient-rich ingredients, it has the potential to enhance the nutritional value of the smoothie and contribute to its overall healthiness.

Recipe for a smoothie cube that helps increase alkalinity.

www.ingramcontent.com/pod-product-compliance
Lightning Source LLC
Chambersburg PA
CBHW051738020426
42333CB00014B/1370